This Journal Belongs to

Published by

Lovely Hearts Publishing

Made in the USA
Coppell, TX
04 December 2024

41775854R00069